How to lose weight in 7 days

Your Ultimate Guide to Achieving Quick and Sustainable Results!

George Brown

TABLE OF CONTENT

Introduction

- Briefly introduce the concept of the eBook.

- Explain the importance of setting realistic expectations.

- Provide an overview of the 7-day weight loss plan.

Chapter 1: Setting the Foundation

- Discuss the importance of a positive mindset.

- Explain the significance of goal setting.

- Introduce the concept of a healthy lifestyle.

Chapter 2: Nutrition for Rapid Weight Loss

- Provide guidance on creating a balanced meal plan.

- Discuss portion control and calorie awareness.

- Include tips for making healthier food choices.

Chapter 3: Effective Workouts for Quick Results

- Explain the benefits of exercise in a short-term weight loss plan.

- Offer a 7-day workout routine that includes cardio and strength training.

- Emphasize the importance of consistency.

Chapter 4: Hydration and Detoxification

- Highlight the role of water in weight loss.

- Discuss the benefits of detoxifying your body.

- Suggest ways to incorporate hydration and detox into the 7-day plan.

Chapter 5: Managing Stress and Sleep

- Explain the impact of stress and lack of sleep on weight loss.

- Offer stress management techniques.

- Provide tips for improving sleep quality.

Chapter 6: Tracking Progress and Staying Motivated

- Discuss the importance of tracking your weight loss journey.

- Offer motivation strategies to stay on track.

- Share success stories and testimonials.

Chapter 7: Safety and Sustainability

- Address the importance of a long-term approach to weight management.

- Provide guidance on transitioning from the 7-day plan to a sustainable lifestyle.

- Highlight the significance of consulting a healthcare professional.

Conclusion

- Summarize key takeaways from the eBook.

- Encourage readers to take action and start their 7-day weight loss journey

Appendix

- Include meal plans, workout routines, and recipes.

- Offer additional tips and resources for Readers

INTRODUCTION

 "How to Lose Weight in 7 Days" – Your Ultimate Guide to Achieving Quick and Sustainable Results!

In a world where wellness is paramount, the quest for effective and efficient weight loss methods has never been more significant. This eBook serves as your trusted companion on a transformative journey towards a healthier, slimmer you. However, before we delve into the specifics of this 7-day weight loss plan, it's crucial to understand the importance of setting realistic expectations.

Embarking on any weight loss journey necessitates a clear understanding that sustainable results require time, dedication, and commitment. While our 7-day plan promises rapid progress, it's essential to remember that achieving lasting change involves more than just a week of effort. This eBook will guide you in harnessing the power of these 7 days to jumpstart your path to a healthier lifestyle, with the understanding that continued effort beyond this timeframe is key.

Now, let's take a sneak peek at what lies ahead in your 7-day weight loss plan. We'll explore a holistic approach encompassing dietary adjustments, exercise routines, and mindfulness practices that work in harmony to help you shed those extra pounds. So, let's get started on your journey towards a healthier, more vibrant you!

Chapter 1: Setting the Foundation

In your quest to lose weight in just 7 days, it's crucial to start with a solid foundation. This chapter lays the groundwork by emphasizing three fundamental principles: the power of a positive mindset, the significance of goal setting, and the introduction to the concept of a healthy lifestyle.

The Power of a Positive Mindset

Before you even take your first step on this journey, it's imperative to recognize the incredible influence your mindset can have on your success. A positive mindset can be your most potent ally when it comes to weight loss. Here's why:

1.1 Embrace Self-Compassion

First and foremost, practice self-compassion. Understand that your journey towards a healthier you may include ups and downs. It's perfectly normal to face challenges along the way. Rather than dwelling on setbacks, treat yourself with kindness and remember that every small effort counts.

1.2 Cultivate Optimism

Optimism fuels motivation. Believe in your ability to achieve your goals, and envision the positive changes that lie ahead. This mental outlook not only boosts your confidence but also keeps you resilient when facing obstacles.

1.3 Banish Negative Self-Talk

Negative self-talk can be a formidable barrier to progress. Identify and challenge those self-defeating thoughts that may be holding you back. Replace them with affirmations that reinforce your commitment to a healthier lifestyle.

The Significance of Goal Setting

Goals are the compass that guides your journey. Setting clear, achievable objectives provides a roadmap for success. Here's how to harness the power of goal setting:

1.4 Set SMART Goals

Make your goals Specific, Measurable, Achievable, Relevant, and Time-bound (SMART). For example, instead of saying, "I want to lose weight," set a goal like, "I aim to lose 5 pounds in the next 7 days by following a balanced diet and exercise plan."

1.5 Break It Down

Divide your long-term weight loss goal into smaller, manageable milestones. These smaller victories will keep you motivated and provide a sense of accomplishment along the way.

1.6 Visualize Success

Immerse yourself in the image of your future self – healthier, more energetic, and confident. Visualization can be a potent tool in helping you stay committed to your goals.

Introducing the Concept of a Healthy Lifestyle

Losing weight in just 7 days is a remarkable goal, but it's essential to view it as the beginning of a lifelong commitment to a healthier lifestyle. This isn't about quick fixes; it's about sustainable change:

1.7 Focus on Holistic Health

Recognize that true health extends beyond the number on the scale. It encompasses physical fitness, mental well-being, and overall quality of life. A healthy lifestyle is about balance and harmony in all these aspects.

1.8 Embrace Nutritional Awareness

Understanding the role of nutrition is pivotal. This eBook will guide you in making informed dietary choices that support your weight loss goals while nourishing your body with essential nutrients.

1.9 Prioritize Physical Activity

Physical activity is a key component of a healthy lifestyle. We'll explore exercise routines that complement your weight loss plan and contribute to your overall well-being.

By embracing these principles of positivity, goal setting, and the broader concept of a healthy lifestyle, you're laying the foundation for a successful 7-day weight loss journey. Remember, it all begins with the right mindset and a clear sense of purpose. In the chapters to come, we'll dive deeper into practical strategies to achieve your goal

Chapter 2:

Nutrition for Rapid Weight Loss

As you embark on your 7-day journey to shed those extra pounds, one of the most critical aspects to consider is nutrition. In this chapter, we'll delve into the essentials of crafting a balanced meal plan, mastering portion control, and developing calorie awareness. Additionally, we'll explore strategies for making healthier food choices that align with your weight loss goals.

Creating a Balanced Meal Plan

A balanced meal plan is the cornerstone of any successful weight loss endeavor. It provides your body with the essential nutrients it needs while helping you achieve your desired results. Here's how to get started:

2.1 Incorporate a Variety of Foods

Diversity is key. Aim to include a wide range of fruits, vegetables, lean proteins, whole grains, and healthy fats in your daily meals. This ensures you receive a broad spectrum of vitamins and minerals.

2.2 Prioritize Lean Proteins

Proteins are your allies in weight loss. They promote satiety and help preserve muscle mass. Opt for lean sources like poultry, fish, tofu, and legumes.

2.3 Choose Whole Grains

Swap refined grains for whole grains like brown rice, quinoa, and whole wheat bread. They provide sustained energy and keep you feeling fuller for longer.

Portion Control and Calorie Awareness

Controlling portion sizes and being aware of your calorie intake are vital aspects of effective weight management. Here's how to approach them:

2.4 Practice Mindful Eating

Slow down during meals and savor each bite. Pay attention to your body's hunger and fullness cues. This mindful approach can help prevent overeating.

2.5 Use Smaller Plates and Bowls

Trick your brain into thinking you're eating more by using smaller dishes. It's a simple yet effective way to control portion sizes.

2.6 Keep a Food Journal

Track your meals and snacks to gain insight into your eating habits. This can help you identify areas where you can make healthier choices and manage your calorie intake more effectively.

Making Healthier Food Choices

To achieve rapid weight loss, it's essential to make informed decisions about what you eat. Here are some practical tips:

2.7 Read Food Labels

Pay attention to food labels, especially when purchasing packaged foods. Look for products with lower levels of added sugars, saturated fats, and sodium.

2.8 Opt for Whole, Unprocessed Foods

Choose foods in their natural state whenever possible. Fresh fruits, vegetables, lean proteins, and whole grains are nutrient-dense and support your weight loss goals.

2.9 Plan Your Meals Ahead

Prepare meals and snacks in advance to avoid impulsive, less healthy choices. Having nutritious options readily available can help you stay on track.

Incorporating these nutrition-focused strategies into your 7-day weight loss plan will set you on the path to success. Remember, it's about nourishing your body while achieving your goals, and with each well-informed choice, you're one step closer to your target weight. In the next chapter, we'll explore the importance of physical activity in accelerating your weight loss journey.

Chapter 3: Effective Workouts for Quick Results

In your quest to lose weight in just 7 days, exercise becomes a crucial ally. This chapter will illuminate the benefits of incorporating physical activity into your short-term weight loss plan, provide you with a 7-day workout routine that combines cardio and strength training, and emphasize the pivotal role of consistency in achieving rapid results.

The Benefits of Exercise in a Short-Term Weight Loss Plan

Exercise offers an array of advantages when pursuing short-term weight loss:

3.1 Accelerated Calorie Burn

Physical activity revs up your metabolism, burning calories even when you're at rest. This can significantly enhance the speed of your weight loss.

3.2 Muscle Preservation

Combining exercise with diet helps preserve lean muscle mass. This is vital because muscle burns more calories than fat, further boosting your metabolism.

3.3 Improved Mood and Energy

Exercise releases endorphins, the body's natural mood boosters, and provides an energy surge. This can be a game-changer, especially during a short-term weight loss program.

Your 7-Day Workout Routine

To maximize your weight loss efforts in just one week, follow this structured workout plan:

Day 1: Cardio Blast

- 30 minutes of brisk walking or jogging

- 10 minutes of bodyweight exercises (push-ups, squats, lunges)

Day 2: Strength and Tone

- 20 minutes of strength training (dumbbell exercises or resistance bands)

- 15 minutes of yoga or stretching

Day 3: High-Intensity Interval Training (HIIT)

- 15 minutes of HIIT workouts (jumping jacks, burpees, mountain climbers)

- 15 minutes of light cardio (walking or cycling)

Day 4: Active Rest

- 30 minutes of low-intensity activity (gentle yoga, easy walking)

- Focus on recovery and relaxation

Day 5: Cardio Intervals

- 30 minutes of alternating between high-intensity and low-intensity cardio (sprinting, walking)

- 10 minutes of core exercises (planks, leg raises)

Day 6: Total Body Workout

- 20 minutes of full-body strength training

- 15 minutes of light cardio or a nature walk

Day 7: Final Push

- 20 minutes of circuit training (combining cardio and strength exercises)

- 10 minutes of deep stretching

The Importance of Consistency

Consistency is the linchpin of any successful weight loss plan. Here's why it matters:

3.4 Building Healthy Habits

Regular exercise establishes a routine, making it easier to adhere to a healthier lifestyle beyond these 7 days.

3.5 Maximizing Results

Consistent workouts optimize calorie burn and muscle development, leading to faster and more sustainable weight loss.

3.6 Boosting Confidence

Achieving your daily workout goals enhances your self-esteem and motivation, reinforcing your commitment to the program.

Incorporate this 7-day workout routine into your weight loss plan with determination and dedication. Remember, it's not just about the week ahead but about setting the stage for long-term success. In the next chapter, we'll delve into strategies to stay motivated and maintain your newfound healthy habits beyond the initial 7 days.

Chapter 4: Hydration and Detoxification

In your journey to lose weight in just 7 days, two often overlooked yet critical components are hydration and detoxification. This chapter will emphasize the pivotal role of water in weight loss, elucidate the benefits of detoxifying your body, and provide practical ways to incorporate hydration and detoxification into your 7-day plan.

The Role of Water in Weight Loss

Water is your body's best friend when it comes to shedding pounds rapidly:

4.1 Appetite Suppression

Drinking water before meals can help you feel fuller, reducing your calorie intake during meals.

4.2 Enhanced Metabolism

Proper hydration ensures your metabolism functions optimally, aiding in calorie burn and fat loss.

4.3 Detoxification

Water helps flush toxins from your body, supporting overall health and aiding in weight loss.

The Benefits of Detoxifying Your Body

Detoxification is a process that can have numerous benefits during your 7-day weight loss journey:

4.4 Improved Digestion

Detoxification can enhance your digestive system, allowing for better absorption of nutrients from the foods you eat.

4.5 Increased Energy

As your body rids itself of harmful substances, you may experience increased energy levels, helping you stay active and motivated.

4.6 Reduced Bloating

Detoxification can alleviate bloating and water retention, contributing to a leaner appearance.

Incorporating Hydration and Detox into the 7-Day Plan

Here are practical ways to make hydration and detoxification a seamless part of your 7-day weight loss plan:

4.7 Set a Hydration Goal

Aim to drink at least 8-10 glasses (64-80 ounces) of water daily. Carry a reusable water bottle to help you track your intake.

4.8 Infuse Your Water

Enhance your hydration by infusing your water with slices of lemon, cucumber, or mint for added flavor and detox benefits.

4.9 Prioritize Herbal Teas

Incorporate herbal teas such as green tea or ginger tea into your daily routine. They not only hydrate but also support detoxification and boost metabolism.

4.10 Consume Water-Rich Foods

Include water-rich foods like watermelon, cucumber, and celery in your meals and snacks. These foods contribute to your daily hydration needs.

4.11 Limit Sugary and Caffeinated Beverages

Reduce or eliminate sugary drinks and excessive caffeine intake, as they can lead to dehydration and disrupt your weight loss efforts.

By focusing on proper hydration and incorporating detoxifying practices into your 7-day plan, you're not only supporting your weight loss goals but also nurturing your overall well-being. In the next chapter, we'll explore strategies for maintaining your newfound health and weight beyond this initial week, ensuring long-term success.

Chapter 5: Managing Stress and Sleep

In your rapid 7-day weight loss journey, it's essential to address two often underestimated factors: stress and sleep. This chapter will delve into the profound impact of stress and inadequate sleep on your weight loss goals, offer effective stress management techniques, and provide valuable tips for enhancing your sleep quality.

The Impact of Stress and Lack of Sleep on Weight Loss

Understanding how stress and insufficient sleep can hinder your weight loss progress is vital:

5.1 Stress and Weight Gain

Chronic stress triggers the release of cortisol, a hormone that can lead to increased appetite and fat storage, making it challenging to shed those extra pounds.

5.2 Sleep and Hormonal Balance

Inadequate sleep disrupts hormonal balance, affecting hunger-regulating hormones like leptin and ghrelin. This can lead to cravings and overeating.

5.3 Energy and Motivation

Both stress and lack of sleep can drain your energy and motivation, making it more challenging to stick to your exercise and diet plan.

Stress Management Techniques

Here are some practical techniques to manage stress effectively during your 7-day weight loss journey:

5.4 Deep Breathing

Practice deep breathing exercises to calm your nervous system. Inhale deeply through your nose for a count of four, hold for four, and exhale slowly through your mouth for a count of six.

5.5 Mindfulness Meditation

Regular mindfulness meditation can reduce stress and increase self-awareness. Spend a few minutes each day in focused meditation to promote relaxation.

5.6 Physical Activity

Exercise is an excellent stress reliever. Incorporate daily physical activity into your routine to release endorphins and reduce stress.

5.7 Time Managements

Efficiently managing your time can reduce stress. Prioritize tasks, set achievable goals, and avoid overloading your schedule.

Tips for Improving Sleep Quality

To ensure you get the restorative sleep your body needs for weight loss, consider these sleep-enhancing strategies:

5.8 Establish a Sleep Routine

Go to bed and wake up at the same time each day to regulate your body's internal clock.

5.9 Create a Relaxing Bedtime Ritual

Engage in calming activities before bed, such as reading, taking a warm bath, or practicing gentle yoga.

5.10 Optimize Your Sleep Environment

Ensure your sleep space is cool, dark, and comfortable. Invest in a supportive mattress and pillows to promote restful sleep.

5.11 Limit Screen Time

Avoid screens like smartphones and laptops before bedtime, as the blue light emitted can disrupt your sleep-wake cycle.

By effectively managing stress and improving your sleep quality, you're creating an environment in which your body can thrive and maximize its weight loss potential. In the final chapter, we'll wrap up your 7-day weight loss journey, offering guidance on transitioning to a sustainable, long-term healthy lifestyle to maintain your success.

Chapter 6: Tracking Progress and Staying Motivated

In this pivotal chapter, we will explore the significance of tracking your weight loss journey, offer effective motivation strategies to keep you on course, and share inspiring success stories and testimonials from individuals who have achieved remarkable results. These insights will empower you to persevere and achieve your own 7-day weight loss goals.

The Importance of Tracking Your Weight Loss Journey

Tracking your progress isn't just a matter of curiosity; it's a critical element of your success:

6.1 Visibility of Achievements

Documenting your progress allows you to see and celebrate your achievements, no matter how small they may seem.

6.2 Accountability

When you track your actions and results, you hold yourself accountable, reinforcing your commitment to your goals.

6.3 Course Correction

Regular tracking enables you to identify what's working and what needs adjustment, helping you refine your approach.

Staying Motivated

Maintaining motivation throughout your weight loss journey is key to your success. Here are strategies to keep your spirits high:

6.4 Set Milestones

Break your long-term goal into smaller, achievable milestones. Celebrate each one to stay motivated.

6.5 Visualize Success

Imagine the future you want to achieve daily. Visualizing your success can boost your determination.

6.6 Reward Yourself

Treat yourself when you reach a milestone. Rewards can be a powerful motivator.

6.7 Find an Accountability Partner

Share your journey with a friend or family member who can support and motivate you.

6.8 Join a Community

Connect with others on similar journeys by participating in weight loss communities or forums for encouragement and inspiration.

Success Stories and Testimonials

Here are a few stories of individuals who have transformed their lives with dedication and determination:

Sarah's Story:

Sarah, a mother of two, lost 10 pounds in her 7-day weight loss journey. She says, "I learned that consistency and self-compassion are keys to success. Even on tough days, I kept going, and it paid off!"

John's Testimonial:

John, a desk worker, achieved remarkable results in just one week. He shares, "Staying active during my lunch break and eating balanced meals made a huge difference. I'm more energized than ever!"

Emily's Journey:

Emily embarked on her 7-day journey with skepticism but emerged a believer. She lost 7 pounds and emphasizes, "The power of mindset and commitment surprised me. Now I know I can achieve anything I set my mind to."

These stories and testimonials are a testament to the transformative potential of your 7-day weight loss plan. Remember, success is within your reach, and the journey may be challenging at times, but the rewards are immeasurable.

As you progress, track your achievements, stay motivated, and draw inspiration from these stories and countless others who have achieved their weight loss goals. Your dedication and determination will carry you through to a healthier, happier you.

With the knowledge, strategies, and support you've gained from this eBook, you're well-equipped to conquer your 7-day weight loss journey and beyond. Stay motivated, stay focused, and let your journey be a source of inspiration for yourself and others. Your success awaits!

Chapter 7: Safety and Sustainability

Congratulations on completing your 7-day weight loss journey! As you bask in the success of your rapid results, it's crucial to shift your focus toward long-term weight management, safety, and sustainability. In this final chapter, we'll address these essential aspects to ensure your newfound health and vitality endure.

The Importance of a Long-Term Approach

While your 7-day journey has delivered remarkable results, sustainable weight management requires a broader perspective:

7.1 Embrace a Lifestyle Change

Recognize that lasting change is not about quick fixes or crash diets. It's about adopting a sustainable, healthy lifestyle that you can maintain over time.

7.2 Gradual Progress

Acknowledge that your weight loss journey may not always be linear. There may be periods of plateaus or even slight setbacks, but these are part of the process.

Transitioning to a Sustainable Lifestyle

Here's how to transition from your 7-day plan to a lifestyle that supports your long-term weight management goals:

7.3 Maintain Healthy Habits

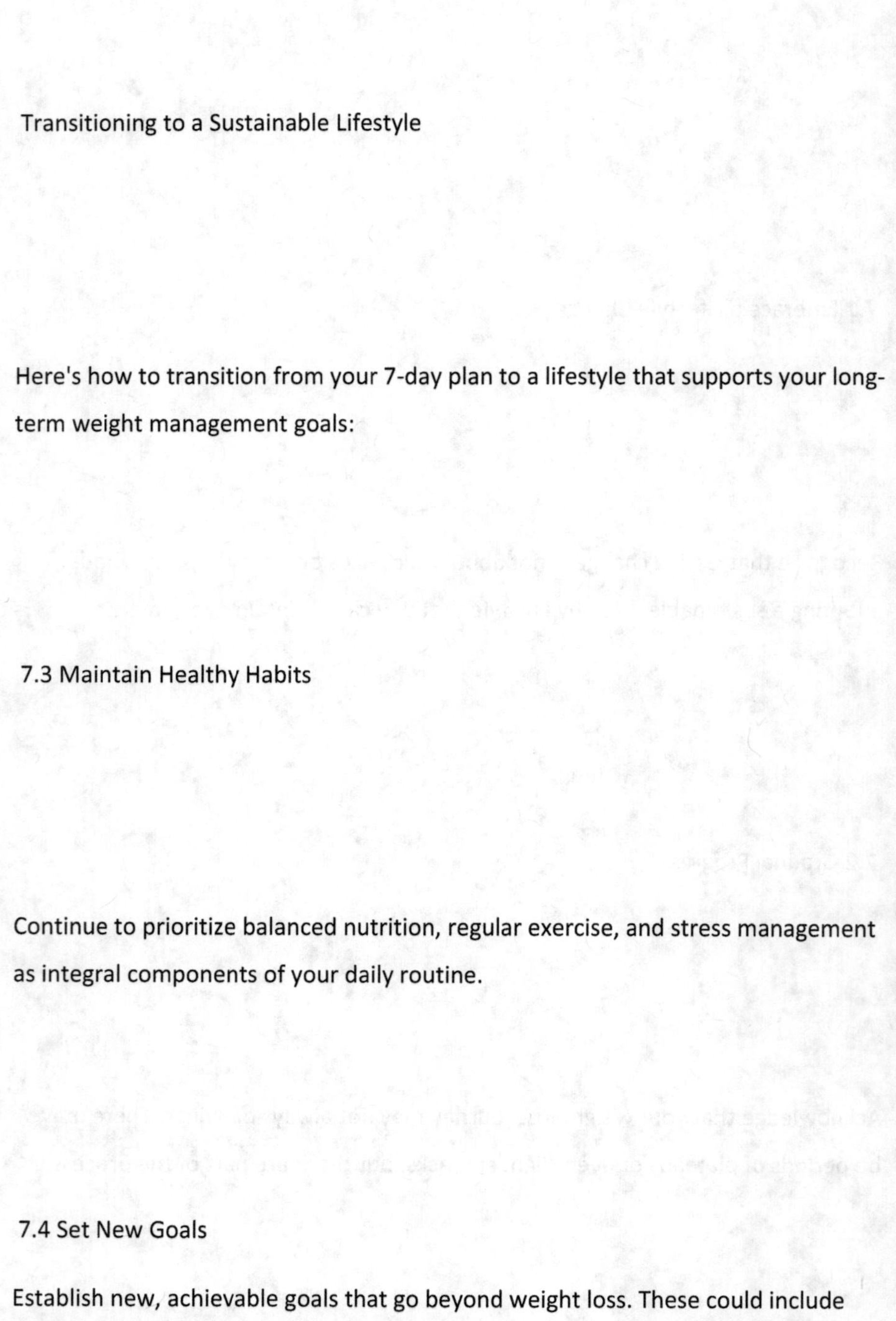

Continue to prioritize balanced nutrition, regular exercise, and stress management as integral components of your daily routine.

7.4 Set New Goals

Establish new, achievable goals that go beyond weight loss. These could include fitness milestones, improved energy levels, or enhanced overall well-being.

7.5 Seek Support

Enlist the support of friends, family, or a weight loss community to stay motivated and accountable in your journey.

 The Significance of Consulting a Healthcare Professional

Before embarking on any weight loss or fitness program, consider the importance of seeking guidance from a healthcare professional:

7.6 Individualized Approach

Consulting with a healthcare provider can help you tailor your weight loss plan to your unique needs, ensuring safety and effectiveness.

7.7 Underlying Health Conditions

A healthcare professional can identify and address any underlying health issues that may affect your weight loss journey.

7.8 Monitoring Progress

Regular check-ins with a healthcare provider can help track your progress, adjust your plan as needed, and provide ongoing support.

Your 7-day weight loss journey has been a remarkable achievement, demonstrating your commitment to a healthier you. By adopting a long-term approach, transitioning to sustainable habits, and consulting a healthcare professional when needed, you're well on your way to maintaining your success and enjoying a lifetime of health and vitality.

Thank you for joining us on this transformative journey. Your dedication to your well-being is a testament to the incredible potential for positive change within us all. We wish you continued success, health, and happiness on your path to long-term weight management.

Conclusion: Your Journey Begins Now

Congratulations on reaching the conclusion of "How to Lose Weight in Seven Days." Throughout this eBook, we've explored the fundamental principles of rapid weight loss and the essentials of a healthier lifestyle. Now, let's recap the key takeaways that will empower you to embark on your own 7-day weight loss journey:

Chapter 1: Setting the Foundation

- Cultivate a positive mindset to stay motivated and resilient.

- Set SMART goals to provide direction and focus.

- Understand that a healthy lifestyle is a long-term commitment.

Chapter 2: Nutrition for Rapid Weight Loss

- Create a balanced meal plan with diverse, nutrient-rich foods.

- Master portion control and calorie awareness for effective weight management.

- Make informed food choices to support your goals.

Chapter 3: Effective Workouts for Quick Results

- Recognize the benefits of exercise in achieving rapid weight loss.

- Follow the 7-day workout routine that combines cardio and strength training.

- Prioritize consistency to maximize your results.

Chapter 4: Hydration and Detoxification

- Embrace the role of water in weight loss and overall health.

- Understand the benefits of detoxifying your body.

- Incorporate hydration and detox practices into your daily routine.

Chapter 5: Managing Stress and Sleep

- Recognize the impact of stress and lack of sleep on weight loss.

- Practice stress management techniques to reduce tension and anxiety.

- Improve sleep quality for optimal physical and mental well-being.

Chapter 7: Safety and Sustainability

- Embrace a long-term approach to weight management and lifestyle change.

- Transition from the 7-day plan to a sustainable, healthy routine.

- Consider consulting a healthcare professional for personalized guidance.

Now, armed with knowledge, determination, and a clear roadmap, it's time to take action. Your 7-day weight loss journey begins today! Remember that every small step you take is a step closer to your goals.

Your success depends on your commitment, consistency, and belief in your ability to make positive changes. Stay focused, stay motivated, and stay true to yourself. The power to transform your life and achieve your weight loss goals is within your grasp.

Don't wait for tomorrow; start your journey today. Your healthier, happier, and more vibrant future is just seven days away. Begin your adventure towards a better you, and let this eBook be your trusted guide along the way.

Appendix: Resources and Tools for Your Success

In this appendix, you'll find valuable resources, including meal plans, workout routines, and recipes, to support your 7-day weight loss journey and beyond. These tools are designed to enhance your experience and provide you with practical guidance for achieving your goals.

7-Day Meal Plans

Here, we've included sample meal plans to assist you in creating balanced, nutritious daily menus that align with your weight loss objectives. These plans can serve as templates for crafting your own meals:

Day 1: Sample Breakfast, Lunch, Dinner, and Snacks

Day 2: Sample Breakfast, Lunch, Dinner, and Snacks

Day 3 Sample Breakfast, Lunch, Dinner, and Snacks

Day 4: Sample Breakfast, Lunch, Dinner, and Snacks

Day 5 Sample Breakfast, Lunch, Dinner, and Snacks

Day 6 Sample Breakfast, Lunch, Dinner, and Snacks

Day 7: Sample Breakfast, Lunch, Dinner, and Snacks

7-Day Workout Routines

We've provided detailed workout routines for each day of your 7-day weight loss plan, combining cardio and strength training exercises to optimize your results. These routines are designed to be adaptable to your fitness level:

Day 1: Cardio Blast and Bodyweight Exercises

Day 2: Strength and Tone with Yoga or Stretching

Day 3: High-Intensity Interval Training (HIIT)

Day 4 Active Rest and Low-Intensity Activity

Day 5 Cardio Intervals and Core Exercises

Day 6.Total Body Workout and Light Cardio

Day 7 Circuit Training and Deep Stretching

Healthy Recipes

Discover a collection of nutritious and delicious recipes that can be incorporated into your meal plan. These recipes are designed to support your weight loss journey while tantalizing your taste buds:

Breakfast: Energizing Smoothie Bowl

Lunch: Grilled Chicken and Quinoa Salad

Dinner: Baked Salmon with Asparagus and Brown Rice

Snacks: Greek Yogurt Parfait and Veggie Sticks with Hummus

Additional Tips and Resources

For further support on your weight loss journey, consider exploring these additional resources and tips:

Online Communities: Join online weight loss communities or forums to connect with like-minded individuals for support, advice, and motivation.

Fitness Apps: Download fitness and nutrition apps to track your progress, monitor your calorie intake, and access workout routines.

Cooking Classes: Enroll in cooking classes or watch online tutorials to expand your culinary skills and prepare healthy, flavorful meals.

Books and Articles: Explore books and articles on nutrition, fitness, and mindfulness to deepen your knowledge and stay inspired.

Professional Guidance: Consider consulting a registered dietitian, personal trainer, or mental health professional for personalized support.

Remember that your weight loss journey is unique to you, and these resources are here to complement your efforts and enhance your experience. Use them as tools to help you achieve your goals and maintain a healthy, balanced lifestyle beyond the initial 7 days.

We wish you continued success, good health, and a brighter future filled with vitality and well-being. You have the knowledge, determination, and support you need to make your weight loss goals a reality. Embrace your journey, and may it lead you to a healthier, happier you!

Best of luck on your 7-day weight loss journey! You've got this!